World Without Women

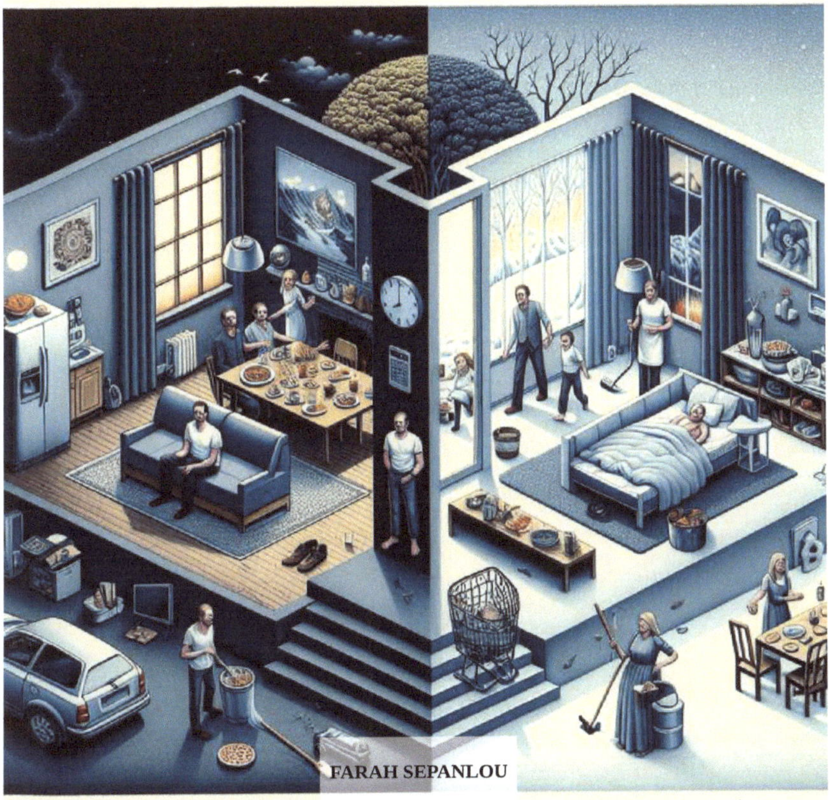

SUMMARY

1

The Simplicity of Men's Lives Without Women

1.1 Daily Routines and Lifestyle Choices

The exploration of men's daily routines and lifestyle choices in the absence of women unveils a stark simplicity that might seem unimaginable to many. This simplicity is not just a matter of preference but rather a reflection of an unadorned approach to life that prioritizes functionality over form, convenience over meticulousness. The essence of this lifestyle can be distilled into several key components, each highlighting how the absence of women could potentially reshape men's lives.

Firstly, personal grooming and cleanliness take on a minimalist approach. Men might find themselves abandoning the routine of shaving and washing regularly, not out of negligence but as a nod to practicality where appearance holds less societal pressure without the influence or expectations from women. This extends to clothing choices, where comfort and utility reign supreme. The typical wardrobe simplifies to essentials like shirts, sweats, socks, and even outdoor shoes that prioritize ease over style.

In terms of domestic life, the kitchen becomes a place less frequented for its traditional purpose. The reliance on kitchen utensils diminishes as disposable dishes become the norm alongside a diet that leans heavily towards convenience foods such as cold cuts and pizza. This shift reflects not only a change in dietary habits but also an alteration in social dining practices that often revolve around family meals prepared and shared together.

- Personal grooming takes a backseat with less emphasis on regular shaving or washing.

- Clothing choices pivot towards comfort and practicality over fashion or occasion-specific attire.

- Kitchen utilities see reduced usage with a marked preference for disposable items and ready-to-eat meals.

The living space itself mirrors this simplicity with minimal furnishings centered around entertainment and basic living needs—a large TV, a refrigerator, and perhaps a vacuum cleaner embody the quintessential items deemed necessary. Such an environment suggests not only physical but also emotional simplicity where attachments to material possessions are minimized.

This exploration into daily routines and lifestyle choices underlines how profoundly women influence men's lives—not just in direct interactions but through societal norms, expectations, and roles that shape behaviors, preferences, and even domestic environments. While this hypothetical scenario paints a picture of extreme simplicity, it also opens up discussions about gender roles, mutual influence, and the complexity hidden within seemingly simple daily choices.

1.2 The Minimalist Approach to Home and Comfort

The minimalist approach to home and comfort, particularly in the context of men living without women, underscores a profound shift towards simplicity and functionality. This lifestyle choice reflects a broader societal trend but is accentuated in scenarios where men opt for or find themselves in solitude. The essence of minimalism here is not just about reducing clutter or owning fewer items; it's deeply rooted in the prioritization of space, time, and resources that align with personal freedom and efficiency.

At the heart of this minimalist approach is the concept of intentional living—choosing to surround oneself with only what is necessary and what brings joy or utility. For many men, this translates into a living space that is devoid of excess furniture, decorations, or kitchenware. A sofa, a bed, a table for eating or working, and essential cooking appliances often constitute the entirety of their domestic setup. This spartan arrangement isn't merely a statement against consumerism; it's a practical response to modern life's complexities, offering an uncluttered environment that promotes focus and tranquility.

The minimalist home extends beyond furniture to include digital spaces as well. Entertainment setups are streamlined with multifunctional devices that serve as both workstations and media centers, reducing the need for multiple gadgets. This integration reflects a holistic view of minimalism as not just physical decluttering but also simplifying one's digital footprint.

- Intentional living through selective ownership
- Spartan yet functional domestic arrangements
- Streamlined entertainment and workspaces

This minimalist approach has significant implications for comfort and well-being. By eliminating unnecessary distractions and possessions, individuals report increased levels of satisfaction with their living conditions. They find more time for hobbies, self-improvement, and relaxation—activities that contribute to mental health and overall happiness. Moreover, this lifestyle fosters a sense of competence in managing one's environment efficiently, leading to greater autonomy and self-reliance.

In conclusion, the minimalist approach to home and comfort among men without women is not merely about austerity or deprivation; it's about creating space for what truly matters. It challenges traditional notions of success measured by material wealth, proposing instead a life enriched by experiences, personal growth, and meaningful connections—even if those connections are primarily with oneself.

1.3 Entertainment Preferences and Social Isolation

The exploration of entertainment preferences among men living without women reveals a nuanced landscape of choices that often leans towards simplicity, yet underscores a complex relationship with social isolation. This preference for straightforward, undemanding forms of entertainment can be seen as an extension of the minimalist lifestyle discussed earlier, but it also opens up a dialogue about the ways in which these choices impact social connections and mental health.

Many men in such situations gravitate towards digital media as a primary source of entertainment, favoring video games, streaming services, and online forums. These platforms not only offer an escape from reality but also provide a sense of community and belonging that might be missing in their offline lives. Video games, for instance, allow for immersive experiences where skills can be honed and achievements unlocked, offering a tangible sense of progress and accomplishment. Streaming services cater to individual tastes with unprecedented precision, ensuring that even the most niche interests are satisfied.

However, this digital-centric approach to entertainment has its drawbacks. The ease of access and the personalized nature of digital content can lead to increased screen time, potentially exacerbating feelings of isolation and loneliness. The paradox here is evident: while these forms of entertainment offer a temporary reprieve from solitude, they can also contribute to its perpetuation by replacing real-world interactions with virtual ones.

- Digital media as both solace and isolator
- Video games providing achievement and community
- Streaming services catering to individual preferences

This dynamic raises important questions about the balance between online engagement and offline socialization. For some men living alone, digital communities may serve as vital support networks that offer companionship and understanding. Yet, there's an ongoing challenge in finding equilibrium between embracing the benefits of these platforms and recognizing when they might be contributing to further social withdrawal.

In conclusion, while the minimalist approach to life may simplify certain aspects of living alone for men without women—streamlining possessions and reducing physical clutter—the realm of entertainment preferences highlights a more complicated picture. It illustrates how simplicity in one area can lead to complexity in another, especially when considering the long-term effects on social connections and mental well-being.

2

The Impact on Family Dynamics

2.1 The Absence of Maternal Influence in Childrearing

The absence of maternal influence in childrearing presents a profound shift in the dynamics of family life, affecting not only the immediate emotional and psychological well-being of children but also their long-term development and socialization. Mothers traditionally play a critical role in nurturing, teaching, and modeling behaviors for their children. Their absence can leave a void that is difficult to fill by other means.

One significant impact of this absence is on the emotional development of children. Mothers often provide a primary source of comfort, security, and understanding for their offspring. Without this maternal presence, children may struggle with forming secure attachments or managing their emotions effectively. This can lead to increased anxiety, depression, and difficulties in forming healthy relationships later in life.

Educationally, mothers frequently serve as the first teachers for their children. They introduce basic concepts such as language, numbers, and social norms. The lack of maternal guidance can hinder cognitive development and academic achievement. Children without strong maternal figures may exhibit delays in speech and language skills, lower academic performance, and reduced motivation to pursue educational opportunities.

- Emotional Support: The unique comfort and security provided by mothers cannot be understated.

- Educational Guidance: Mothers play a crucial role in early learning experiences.

- Social Development: Maternal influence significantly affects children's ability to navigate social interactions.

In terms of socialization, mothers often facilitate early social interactions and teach important skills such as empathy, cooperation, and conflict resolution. The absence of these lessons can result in children experiencing challenges with peer relationships and adapting to societal expectations. Furthermore, maternal figures typically model gender roles within the family context; without this example, children might struggle with understanding or accepting diverse gender identities and expressions.

While it is essential to recognize that fathers and other caregivers can provide loving support and guidance to children effectively overcoming many hurdles associated with the absence of a mother's influence requires concerted effort from the entire support network surrounding a child. This includes extended family members, educators, healthcare providers, and community organizations all playing pivotal roles in ensuring that children receive the comprehensive care they need for healthy development.

In conclusion, while families come in all forms and are capable of providing love and support through various structures, the specific contributions made by mothers are uniquely valuable. Addressing the gap left by an absent maternal figure demands awareness of these impacts alongside proactive strategies to mitigate them—ensuring every child has access to the nurturing environment necessary for thriving physically, emotionally, and socially.

2.2 Challenges in Nurturing and Emotional Support

The nurturing process and provision of emotional support are critical components of child development, deeply influencing a child's emotional health, self-esteem, and social competencies. However, various factors can significantly challenge the effectiveness of these essential parenting roles. This section delves into the complexities surrounding nurturing practices and the provision of emotional support, highlighting key challenges that families may encounter.

One primary challenge is the evolving structure of family units. In contemporary society, single-parent households, blended families, and other non-traditional family structures have become more common. While these families can provide loving and supportive environments, they may also face unique stressors such as financial strain, societal stigma, or logistical complications in coordinating care and attention among multiple guardians. These stressors can inadvertently affect the quality and consistency of nurturing and emotional support provided to children.

Additionally, the increasing demands of modern life pose a significant challenge. Many parents find themselves balancing work commitments with family responsibilities, leading to time constraints that limit their availability for one-on-one interactions with their children. This scarcity of quality time can hinder opportunities for meaningful conversations, shared experiences, and the development of a deep emotional bond between parent and child.

- Economic pressures: Financial instability or poverty can exacerbate stress within the household, affecting parents' ability to create a nurturing environment.

- Mental health issues: Parents struggling with their mental health may find it difficult to provide consistent emotional support to their children.

- Cultural differences: Families navigating cross-cultural dynamics may encounter challenges in aligning traditional nurturing practices with those of their surrounding community.

Moreover, digital technology's pervasive influence introduces another layer of complexity. While offering educational benefits and connectivity, excessive screen time can disrupt family interactions and diminish face-to-face communication skills among children. Parents must navigate the delicate balance between leveraging technology for its advantages while mitigating its potential to impede personal connections within the family.

In conclusion, while nurturing and providing emotional support are pivotal to healthy child development, modern families face multifaceted challenges in fulfilling these roles effectively. Addressing these issues requires awareness, flexibility in parenting approaches, and seeking external support when necessary—ensuring that all children receive the love and guidance needed to thrive emotionally and socially.

2.3 A World Devoid of Motherly Love and Care

The absence of motherly love and care in a child's life marks a profound deficit, impacting not just the emotional but also the psychological development of the individual. This section explores the ramifications of such an absence, delving into how it shapes a person's ability to form relationships, self-perceive, and navigate societal norms. The nurturing touch of a mother or a mother figure plays an indispensable role in fostering security, empathy, and resilience among children.

Without this foundational support system, children often struggle with issues of trust and attachment. The bond formed through consistent nurturing acts as a blueprint for future relationships; its absence can lead to difficulties in forming healthy attachments or understanding social cues. Moreover, the lack of maternal affection can severely dent self-esteem and confidence, leaving individuals questioning their worth and capabilities.

Academically and socially, children deprived of maternal care may exhibit delays or regressions. They might struggle with academic performance due to a lack of encouragement or face challenges in social integration. Emotional regulation is another area significantly affected by the absence of motherly love. Without having been modeled appropriate ways to express and manage emotions, these individuals may either withdraw emotionally or display heightened aggression.

- Increased susceptibility to mental health issues: Anxiety, depression, and other mental health disorders are more prevalent among those who lacked maternal nurturing during their formative years.

- Risk-taking behaviors: A void left by absent maternal affection can lead individuals to seek fulfillment through substance abuse or unhealthy relationships.

- Challenges in parenting: Without positive models of caregiving from their own upbringing, individuals may find themselves at a loss when faced with parenting responsibilities later in life.

In conclusion, the impact of growing up without motherly love extends far beyond childhood, affecting every facet of personal development and social interaction. It underscores the importance of providing supportive structures for children lacking this essential component—be it through extended family members stepping in as caregivers or through community support systems designed to mitigate these deficits. Recognizing the depth of influence maternal care has on an individual's life trajectory highlights the critical need for interventions aimed at filling this gap wherever possible.

3

Societal Implications of a World Without Women

3.1 Alterations in Professional Fields and Workplaces

The hypothetical absence of women from the world would precipitate profound alterations in professional fields and workplaces, reshaping the very fabric of industries and employment practices. This scenario invites us to consider not just the quantitative loss of half the workforce, but also the qualitative impact on innovation, emotional intelligence, and diversity of thought.

Firstly, sectors traditionally dominated by women, such as healthcare, education, and social services, would face unprecedented challenges. The nurturing roles often associated with nursing or teaching are not merely a matter of staffing numbers but involve qualities and approaches that enrich these professions. Without women, these fields might struggle to maintain their ethos and effectiveness, potentially leading to a depersonalization of care and education.

In contrast, STEM fields (Science, Technology, Engineering, Mathematics), already grappling with gender disparity issues, might see a stagnation in efforts towards diversity and inclusion. The absence of women's perspectives could lead to a narrowing of research focuses and innovation pathways. For instance, studies have shown that female scientists are more likely to engage in research with direct social impact. Their absence could skew research priorities away from holistic solutions addressing wide-ranging societal needs.

- Impact on Healthcare: A decline in empathetic patient care and potential shortages in professions like nursing and mental health counseling.

- Education Sector Challenges: Reduced emphasis on inclusive education strategies and possible declines in educational quality due to lack of diverse teaching methodologies.

- STEM Innovation Stagnation: A slowdown in diversification efforts within STEM fields leading to narrower research outcomes.

Beyond specific sectors, the overall workplace culture would undergo significant shifts. The collaborative dynamics often encouraged by female participation might give way to more hierarchical structures traditionally favored in male-dominated environments. This could affect team cohesion, communication styles, and conflict resolution methods across all industries.

In conclusion, envisioning a world without women compels us to recognize their indispensable contributions across all professional fields. It underscores not only the importance of gender diversity for economic reasons but also for fostering innovative thinking and compassionate service delivery that benefits society as a whole.

3.2 The Cultural Void in Arts, Literature, and Media

The absence of women from the world would not only disrupt professional fields and workplaces but also create a profound cultural void in arts, literature, and media. This section delves into the ramifications of such a scenario, exploring how it would reshape our cultural landscape and expression. Women have historically been both muses and creators in these domains, offering unique perspectives that enrich our collective human experience.

Firstly, the visual arts would lose a significant portion of their diversity and depth. Female artists bring distinct viewpoints to the exploration of themes such as identity, body politics, and social justice. Their absence would mean a loss of nuanced interpretations and expressions in art forms ranging from painting to digital media. Moreover, the representation of women by male artists cannot fully substitute for self-representation by women themselves, leading to a one-dimensional portrayal of female experiences and identities.

In literature, the impact would be equally devastating. Women authors have contributed some of the most critical works in literary history, offering insights into society's fabric through novels, poetry, essays, and memoirs. Their narratives often challenge patriarchal structures and explore complex relationships with an emotional depth that is vital for a holistic understanding of human nature. Without these voices, literature would become monolithic, lacking the rich tapestry woven by diverse gender perspectives.

The realm of media—encompassing film, television, music, and online content—would also suffer greatly. Female directors, writers, actors, and musicians play crucial roles in shaping media narratives that reflect societal values and aspirations. Their creative visions help challenge stereotypes and foster empathy among diverse audiences. A world devoid of women's contributions to media would likely revert to reinforcing traditional gender roles and miss out on stories that challenge societal norms or inspire change.

Furthermore, without women's influence in arts criticism and curation roles—such as editors, gallery owners, producers—the dissemination and interpretation of creative works would narrow significantly. This shift could lead to a homogenization of cultural products available to society at large.

In conclusion,

the absence of women from arts,*literature*,**and media**would not only result in a quantitative reduction in creators but also lead to a qualitative impoverishment of culture itself. The diversity of thought,perspectives,and emotions brought forth by women across these fields is indispensable for a vibrant,*society*. Thus,**recognizing**and valuing female contributions is essential for maintaining the richness*of our collective cultural heritage.*

3.3 Shifts in Social Norms and Interpersonal Relationships

The hypothetical absence of women from the world would precipitate profound shifts in social norms and interpersonal relationships, fundamentally altering the fabric of society. This scenario, while extreme, serves to underscore the integral role women play not only in the professional and cultural spheres but also in shaping social interactions and norms. The dynamics of friendships, family structures, romantic relationships, and even casual interactions would undergo significant transformations.

Firstly, the structure of families would be radically changed. In a world without women, traditional family units based on heterosexual partnerships would no longer exist. This would necessitate a redefinition of family that moves away from biological ties towards more socially constructed networks. Parenting roles would have to be reimagined, potentially leading to a greater acceptance and normalization of diverse family models including single parenthood by choice or necessity and communal parenting arrangements.

In terms of friendships and social bonds, men might develop deeper emotional connections with each other in the absence of women. With societal expectations around masculinity possibly shifting due to these changes, expressions of vulnerability and emotional support among men could become more normalized. This could lead to richer interpersonal relationships among men but might also highlight the void left by the unique emotional support systems often provided by women.

Romantic relationships would also face foundational changes. Without women, individuals who are attracted exclusively to women might struggle with their sexual identities or seek alternative forms of companionship and intimacy. This could lead to an expansion in how society defines romance and intimacy beyond gendered norms.

Moreover, societal norms around gender roles could either become more rigid or begin to dissolve entirely as society adapts to this new reality. Without women to contrast against male behaviors, what is considered "masculine" or "feminine" might shift dramatically over time. This could result in a more homogenous culture where behaviors are less tied to gender expectations or lead to the emergence of new forms of identity expression altogether.

In conclusion, while it is impossible to predict all the ways in which interpersonal relationships and social norms would change in a world without women, it is clear that their absence would leave an indelible mark on society. Women's contributions to fostering empathy, nurturing familial bonds, challenging societal norms through feminist perspectives, and enriching social interactions are irreplaceable components of human civilization.

4

Psychological Consequences on Individuals and Communities

4.1 Emotional Well-being and Mental Health Concerns

The exploration of emotional well-being and mental health concerns is crucial in understanding the broader psychological consequences on individuals and communities. This area delves into the intricate ways in which our mental health is intertwined with our daily lives, societal expectations, and personal experiences. Emotional well-being is not merely the absence of mental illness but encompasses a positive state of mind, where an individual can cope with normal life stresses, work productively, and contribute to their community.

Mental health concerns have been on the rise globally, exacerbated by various factors including economic uncertainties, social isolation, and the stress of modern living. The stigma surrounding mental health issues further complicates individuals' willingness to seek help, leading to a silent crisis that affects millions worldwide. Understanding the multifaceted nature of emotional well-being and mental health concerns requires a comprehensive approach that considers biological, psychological, and social factors.

Moreover, societal changes have introduced new challenges to mental health that were less prevalent in past generations. The digital age has brought about a unique set of pressures related to social media use, online bullying, and the erosion of privacy. These issues highlight the need for updated approaches to mental health education and intervention that are relevant to today's societal context.

- The impact of chronic stress on mental health cannot be overstated. Prolonged exposure to stressors can lead to serious health problems such as depression, anxiety, heart disease, and even memory impairment.

- Social support systems play a critical role in maintaining emotional well-being. Strong relationships with family members, friends, or community groups provide emotional support that can buffer against life's challenges.

- The role of lifestyle factors in influencing mental health is increasingly recognized. Physical activity, diet, sleep patterns, and exposure to nature all have significant effects on emotional well-being.

In conclusion, addressing emotional well-being and mental health concerns requires a holistic strategy that includes raising awareness about mental health issues; promoting healthy lifestyle choices; fostering strong support networks; implementing effective policies at governmental levels; and ensuring access to professional help when needed. By tackling these areas comprehensively we can hope to mitigate some of the adverse effects these issues have on individuals' lives and society as a whole.

4.2 The Role of Women in Fostering Community and Belonging

The role of women in fostering community and belonging is a multifaceted subject that touches upon various aspects of societal development and emotional well-being. Historically, women have been the cornerstone of social cohesion within communities, often leading efforts to nurture connections, support networks, and collective identity. This section delves into how women contribute to the fabric of communities, highlighting their unique approaches to creating spaces of inclusion and mutual support.

Women's contribution to community life can be seen in diverse contexts, from family units to professional environments and broader societal structures. They often initiate and maintain social bonds that are crucial for emotional support and resilience against life's challenges. Through organizing social gatherings, participating in volunteer work, or leading local initiatives, women create opportunities for individuals to connect, share experiences, and foster a sense of belonging.

- Women's roles as caregivers not only strengthen family ties but also model compassion and empathy within the community.

- In many cultures, women are at the forefront of preserving traditions, languages, and cultural practices that are essential for communal identity.

- Through participation in education and local governance, women advocate for inclusive policies that address the needs of diverse community members.

Beyond these traditional roles, modern dynamics have seen women breaking barriers in various sectors while still emphasizing community building. In the professional realm, female leaders often prioritize corporate social responsibility and workplace cultures that value diversity and inclusion. Their approach to leadership frequently incorporates emotional intelligence with an emphasis on collaboration over competition—a style that promotes a sense of belonging among employees.

Furthermore, through digital platforms, women have expanded their influence by creating online communities where individuals find support on issues ranging from parenting to career development. These virtual spaces not only provide information but also foster connections across geographical boundaries.

In conclusion, the role of women in fostering community and belonging is indispensable. Their innate ability to nurture relationships coupled with their leadership in advocating for inclusive practices enriches societal cohesion. By recognizing and supporting the contributions of women in this domain, communities can become more resilient, inclusive, and connected.

4.3 Loss of Diversity in Perspectives and Innovation

The significance of diversity in perspectives and innovation cannot be overstated, as it plays a crucial role in the development and progression of societies, industries, and global markets. This section explores the psychological consequences that arise from a lack of diversity, particularly focusing on how homogeneity can stifle creativity, innovation, and the overall growth within communities and organizations.

Diversity is not just about including different genders, races, or cultures; it's about valuing different ways of thinking, problem-solving approaches, and creative insights that come from varied life experiences. When diversity is lacking, there's a tendency for groupthink to prevail, where conformity overrules critical analysis and dissenting opinions. This environment discourages individuals from proposing unique solutions or challenging the status quo, leading to stagnation.

From an organizational perspective, companies that fail to embrace diversity often find themselves lagging behind in innovation. They are less likely to understand the needs of a global customer base or to create products that appeal to diverse groups. Moreover, without diverse leadership, businesses risk overlooking potential market opportunities that could have been identified through a broader lens of experiences.

- Lack of diversity limits understanding and empathy across cultural divides, reducing the effectiveness of communication within multinational teams.

- Homogeneous groups are more prone to overlooking biases in decision-making processes, which can lead to flawed outcomes.

- A narrow range of perspectives can diminish the capacity for creative problem-solving, making it harder for organizations to adapt during times of change or crisis.

In contrast, communities and organizations that prioritize diversity benefit from a richer tapestry of ideas and viewpoints. Such environments foster innovation by encouraging the cross-pollination of thoughts and concepts across different disciplines and cultures. This not only leads to more effective problem-solving but also enhances adaptability by preparing teams to tackle unforeseen challenges with a multifaceted approach.

In conclusion, the loss of diversity in perspectives significantly undermines innovation and growth within any community or organization. It restricts the pool of ideas available for development projects or strategic initiatives while also diminishing resilience against external pressures. By actively promoting inclusivity and ensuring diverse voices are heard and valued at all levels—whether in community settings or corporate boardrooms—societies can unlock their full potential for progress and innovation.

5

Reimagining Gender Roles and Responsibilities

5.1 Exploring the Significance of Female Contributions

The exploration of female contributions across various spheres of life reveals a profound impact on societal development, cultural richness, and economic growth. Women's roles, traditionally confined to domestic spheres, have evolved dramatically, showcasing their multifaceted contributions beyond the household. This section delves into the significance of these contributions, highlighting how they reshape our understanding of gender roles and responsibilities.

Historically, women have been pivotal in nurturing and maintaining family structures, often seen as the backbone of familial support systems. Their roles as caregivers and educators within the family unit have laid foundational values and principles that shape future generations. However, to view women's contributions solely through this lens would be an oversimplification of their vast potential and achievements.

The significance of female contributions extends beyond tangible achievements; it lies also in challenging traditional gender norms and inspiring future generations to pursue their passions irrespective of societal expectations. The narrative shift from viewing women merely as supporters to recognizing them as leaders in their own right is crucial for achieving gender equality. As we continue to acknowledge and celebrate female contributions across all facets of life, we pave the way for a more equitable world where every individual has the opportunity to thrive based on merit rather than gender.

- Women's participation in the workforce has been a game-changer for economies around the world. From leadership positions to entrepreneurial ventures, women have proven their mettle in driving innovation and fostering economic growth.

- In fields such as science, technology, engineering, and mathematics (STEM), women have made groundbreaking discoveries that challenge gender stereotypes and pave the way for more inclusive representation in these critical areas.

- The arts and literature are replete with examples of female artists, writers, and performers who have enriched cultural landscapes with their unique perspectives and creativity.

- In social justice movements, women have been at the forefront advocating for rights and reforms that benefit not only themselves but society at large. Their resilience in fighting for equality has led to significant legal and societal changes worldwide.

In conclusion, exploring the significance of female contributions offers a richer understanding of humanity's collective achievements. It underscores the necessity of dismantling barriers that hinder women's full participation in all aspects of life. By doing so, we not only honor those who have paved the way but also inspire continued progress towards an inclusive society where everyone can contribute their best without bias or limitation.

5.2 Redefining Masculinity in the Absence of Femininity

The concept of masculinity has traditionally been constructed in opposition to femininity, with societal norms dictating specific roles and behaviors as inherently male or female. However, the evolving understanding of gender as a spectrum rather than a binary necessitates a reevaluation of masculinity independent of its contrast to femininity. This section explores how masculinity can be redefined when it is not defined in opposition to or absence of femininity, offering insights into a more inclusive and nuanced understanding of gender roles.

Redefining masculinity involves dismantling long-standing stereotypes that associate maleness with dominance, aggression, and emotional stoicism. In the absence of these traditional markers, which often rely on a direct contrast to femininity (perceived as submissive, passive, and emotionally expressive), masculinity can embrace qualities traditionally categorized as feminine without loss of identity. This shift allows for a broader range of expressions within masculinity that includes vulnerability, empathy, and nurturing—traits that are beneficial for individuals and society alike.

- Emphasizing emotional intelligence and communication skills as components of a modern masculine identity challenges the notion that men must remain stoic or emotionally distant.

- Promoting active fatherhood and equal participation in domestic responsibilities showcases that caregiving is not inherently feminine but a human quality.

- Encouraging collaboration over competition in professional settings fosters environments where success is not predicated on traditionally masculine traits like assertiveness at the expense of cooperation.

This redefinition does not negate the existence or value of traditionally masculine traits but rather expands the concept to include a wider range of human experiences. It acknowledges that all individuals have the capacity for both 'masculine' and 'feminine' traits, freeing them from restrictive norms that dictate behavior based on gender. Ultimately, redefining masculinity in this way promotes healthier relationships with oneself and others by allowing individuals to express their identities more fully and authentically.

In conclusion, redefining masculinity in the absence of femininity offers an opportunity to construct a more inclusive understanding of gender roles. By embracing qualities across the gender spectrum, society can move towards eliminating harmful stereotypes and fostering environments where everyone is free to express their true selves without constraint. This evolution benefits not only men but all individuals by creating spaces where compassion, empathy, and vulnerability are valued traits in every person regardless of gender.

5.3 Potential for Gender Equality and Shared Duties

The potential for achieving gender equality and shared duties within society is a critical aspect of reimagining gender roles and responsibilities. This vision encompasses a future where tasks, obligations, and opportunities are not dictated by one's gender but are equally accessible and distributed among all individuals, regardless of their gender identity. The realization of this potential requires a multifaceted approach, including the dismantling of traditional gender norms, promoting inclusivity in all spheres of life, and fostering an environment where shared responsibilities are not only encouraged but also valued.

At the heart of this transformative journey is the need to challenge and redefine societal perceptions that have historically placed men and women into rigid categories with specific roles. By advocating for a model of shared duties, we can begin to dismantle the barriers that prevent individuals from pursuing roles or responsibilities traditionally associated with another gender. This shift not only liberates individuals from restrictive stereotypes but also promotes a more balanced distribution of labor both in domestic settings and the workplace.

- Encouraging paternity leave alongside maternity leave as a normative practice underscores the importance of caregiving as a shared responsibility rather than solely a woman's duty.

- Implementing policies that promote work-life balance for all genders ensures that career advancement does not come at the expense of family or personal time, making it easier for both men and women to participate equally in domestic tasks.

- Education plays a pivotal role in shaping future generations' perceptions of gender roles. Integrating discussions on gender equality and shared duties into educational curriculums can foster early awareness and acceptance among children.

In conclusion, the potential for gender equality and shared duties represents not just an idealistic goal but a necessary evolution towards more inclusive societies. By embracing this potential, we pave the way for future generations to live in a world where their abilities define them, not their gender—a world where everyone has equal opportunities to contribute to society fully.

This envisioned future where gender equality and shared duties are realized offers numerous benefits, including stronger familial bonds through active co-parenting, more equitable workplaces that value diversity and collaboration, and societies where every individual has the freedom to choose their path without being constrained by outdated norms. Achieving this potential requires concerted efforts across various sectors—governmental policies must support equal opportunities; workplaces need to adopt flexible practices that accommodate diverse needs; education systems should advocate for inclusivity from an early age; and media representation must challenge stereotypes rather than perpetuate them.

6

The Importance of Women in Society

6.1 Empowering Women in Leadership Roles

The empowerment of women in leadership roles is not just a matter of social justice or equality; it's a catalyst for broader societal change and economic growth. When women ascend to leadership positions, they bring diverse perspectives, innovative approaches, and a focus on inclusive policies that benefit everyone. The importance of empowering women in such roles cannot be overstated, as it challenges the traditional gender norms and paves the way for future generations to envision a world where leadership is defined by capability rather than gender.

One significant aspect of empowering women in leadership is breaking the glass ceiling that has historically limited their rise in various sectors, including politics, business, and academia. Despite progress, women are still underrepresented at the highest levels of decision-making. This underrepresentation is not just a loss for women but for society as a whole, as diverse leadership has been shown to lead to better outcomes in governance, innovation, and problem-solving.

- Creating supportive networks that offer mentorship and sponsorship opportunities for aspiring female leaders.

- Implementing policies that ensure equal pay for equal work and challenge discriminatory practices that hinder women's career advancement.

- Promoting work-life balance through flexible working hours and parental leave policies that enable both men and women to share domestic responsibilities without sacrificing their career goals.

To further empower women in leadership roles, it's crucial to address the systemic barriers they face from an early age. Education plays a pivotal role here; by encouraging girls to pursue studies in traditionally male-dominated fields like STEM (Science, Technology, Engineering, Mathematics), we can gradually increase the pool of qualified women ready to take on leadership roles across all sectors. Additionally, highlighting successful female leaders as role models can inspire young girls to aspire towards leadership positions themselves.

In conclusion, empowering women in leadership roles benefits not only the individuals involved but society at large. It leads to more inclusive decision-making processes and innovative solutions to complex problems. By investing in policies and practices that support gender diversity at the top levels of power, we can build a more equitable world where everyone has the opportunity to lead and succeed.

6.2 Promoting Gender Equality in Education and Career Opportunities

The pursuit of gender equality in education and career opportunities is a cornerstone for achieving a balanced and fair society. This initiative not only addresses the disparities faced by women but also unlocks a wealth of untapped potential, driving innovation and economic growth. By ensuring equal access to educational resources, encouraging participation in diverse fields of study, and dismantling barriers to career advancement, societies can foster an environment where both men and women can thrive equally.

Education serves as the foundation for empowering women with the knowledge, skills, and confidence needed to pursue their ambitions. Historically, gender biases have skewed enrollment in certain disciplines—most notably in STEM (Science, Technology, Engineering, Mathematics) fields—where women are significantly underrepresented. Addressing these imbalances requires targeted interventions such as scholarships for female students, mentorship programs connecting them with successful women in these fields, and curriculum reforms that challenge stereotypes and encourage diversity of thought.

- Implementing policies that promote gender-sensitive teaching methods and materials.
- Creating platforms for showcasing female role models in various careers to inspire young girls.
- Ensuring that career guidance programs are inclusive and support girls' ambitions across all sectors.

In the realm of career opportunities, achieving gender equality means removing systemic barriers that hinder women's progress. Despite advancements towards workplace equality, issues like the gender pay gap, unequal representation in leadership roles, and discrimination continue to persist. Proactive measures such as enforcing equal pay legislation, offering leadership training programs for women, and adopting flexible work arrangements can help bridge these gaps. Moreover, fostering a corporate culture that values diversity and inclusion is crucial for creating environments where everyone has the opportunity to succeed based on merit.

To truly promote gender equality in education and career opportunities, it is essential to engage all stakeholders—including governments, educational institutions, corporations, and civil society—in collaborative efforts. By championing policies that support equal access to education and employment for women, societies can unlock their full potential leading to sustainable development and prosperity for all.

6.3 Celebrating Women's Contributions to Science, Technology, Engineering, and Mathematics (STEM)

The celebration of women's contributions to STEM is not just an act of recognition but a fundamental step towards redefining the future landscape of these fields. Women have historically been underrepresented in STEM, yet their achievements have been pivotal in pushing the boundaries of knowledge and innovation. This section delves into the significance of acknowledging and celebrating female pioneers and contemporaries in STEM, exploring how their visibility can inspire future generations and contribute to a more inclusive scientific community.

Highlighting women's achievements in STEM serves multiple purposes. Firstly, it challenges the prevailing stereotypes that often discourage girls from pursuing careers in these fields. By showcasing successful women scientists, engineers, mathematicians, and technologists, we provide tangible role models for young girls who aspire to enter these disciplines. The stories of trailblazers like Marie Curie, Ada Lovelace, Katherine Johnson, and contemporary figures such as Fei-Fei Li or Gitanjali Rao resonate with potential and possibility.

- Creating awards and recognitions specifically for women in STEM to highlight their contributions and achievements.

- Organizing conferences and seminars that focus on the work of female scientists and engineers.

- Developing educational programs that include comprehensive studies about women's historical contributions to science and technology.

Beyond individual recognition, celebrating women's contributions to STEM encourages institutional change. It prompts academic institutions and corporations to evaluate their policies regarding gender equality, mentorship opportunities, and career advancement for women. This reflection can lead to more supportive environments that not only attract but also retain female talent in STEM fields. Furthermore, public acknowledgment of women's achievements in science and technology acts as a catalyst for cultural change by normalizing female success in traditionally male-dominated arenas.

In conclusion, celebrating women's contributions to STEM is crucial for fostering diversity and driving innovation within these fields. By honoring past accomplishments and supporting current endeavors of women in science and technology, society can move closer towards achieving gender equality in education and career opportunities. This not only benefits aspiring female scientists but enriches the global scientific community by ensuring a diverse range of perspectives are represented in tackling some of the world's most challenging problems.

The book "World Without Women" delves into a speculative scenario where women no longer exist, exploring the profound impact this would have on society, culture, and individual lives. It presents a stark vision of a world simplified to the bare necessities from a male perspective, where cleanliness, grooming, and culinary efforts are minimized to basic levels. The narrative suggests that without women, men would lead simpler lives characterized by rudimentary home environments consisting only of essential appliances and limited entertainment options focused on news and sports.

However, the book goes beyond these surface-level changes to examine deeper societal and emotional voids that would emerge in a world devoid of women. It highlights the absence of maternal warmth, love, and care, emphasizing how crucial women are in nurturing and supporting not just their own children but society at large. The text argues that men cannot replicate the unique roles that women play as mothers, partners, and caretakers.

Moreover, "World Without Women" reflects on the broader implications of such a world on professions traditionally dominated by women—like nursing or teaching—and creative fields where women contribute significantly as artists, writers, and more. It posits that without women's influence and participation in these areas, society would lose out on essential perspectives and talents.

In essence, the book serves as a poignant reminder of the indispensable role of women in shaping a balanced, compassionate, and vibrant world. It challenges readers to appreciate the myriad ways in which women enrich our lives personally and collectively. Through its exploration of a hypothetical world without women, it underscores the value of gender diversity and the irreplaceable contributions of women to all aspects of human life.

www.ingramcontent.com/pod-product-compliance
Lightning Source LLC
Chambersburg PA
CBHW040315240726
48664CB00006B/1500